THE
SUGAR
SEDUCTION

TRINA WIGGINS, MD

Published by Opt2bfit.

Publishing coordination and book design by ELOHAI International Publishing & Media: elohaipublishing.com.

For inquiries or to request bulk copies,

e\mail trinawigginsmdnv@gmail.com.

ISBN: 978-1-953535-59-7

Printed in the United States of America

Table of Contents

Introduction 5
Why is sugar so dangerous? 7
Tips for Dining Out 11

Applebee's 14
Bonefish Grill 15
Boston Market 16
BJ's Restaurant 17
Cheesecake Factory 18
Chick-fil-A 19
Chili's 20
Cracker Barrel 21
Golden Corral 22
Jack in the Box 23
KFC 24
McDonald's 25
Olive Garden 26
Outback Steakhouse 27
Panda Express 28
Panera Bread 29
Red Lobster 30
Subway 31
Taco Bell 32
Wendy's 33
Yard House 34

About the Author 35
Endnotes 37
Connect and Share 43

Introduction

Let's talk about how sugar stealthily infiltrates your life and wreaks havoc on your body. Sugar's seduction begins with our young children. While practicing pediatrics in Las Vegas, the majority of my patients reported having a cinnamon roll for breakfast provided by their school. A classic cinnamon roll from Cinnabon has a whopping 61 grams of sugar, more than double the maximum daily amount for women (see American Heart Association recommendations on page 8). I also witnessed young children in the waiting room drinking sodas. Just one 12-ounce can of Coca-Cola contains 39 grams of sugar, which is similarly well above the daily allotment. From these examples, it's no surprise the American Heart Association has found that the average American consumes about 60 pounds of sugar every year.

How did we get here? Well, 74% of packaged food sold in US grocery stores has added sugars, according to sugarscience.ucsf.edu. Many people resort to prepackaged, processed foods for most meals and are unaware that added sugar hides out in a surprising number of foods.

I have had many patients say, "I don't eat cookies, donuts, or other sweets." The unfortunate reality is that sugar is not only found in sweet goods. It can also be found in breakfast cereals, yogurt, alcoholic beverages, and condiments like barbecue sauces, teriyaki sauces, salad dressings, and ketchup.

Since not all sugar is sweet, it is vitally important to read food labels to monitor your consumption of added sugars. Be aware that the food industry has disguised sugar in a variety of names such as corn sweetener, agave nectar, beet sugar, brown rice syrup, honey, dehydrated cane juice, maltodextrin, malt syrup, sorghum, fruit juice concentrate, high-fructose corn syrup, invert sugar, molasses, dextrose, fructose, glucose, lactose, maltose, sucralose, and sucrose.

It takes only a single bite of sugar to stimulate the brain to release dopamine, a natural chemical that drives our cravings. We interpret this dopamine signal as pleasure, and once the brain senses pleasure, its programming changes to want more. It is this same chemical that causes alcoholics and drug addicts to constantly seek their next high. In fact, research has shown sugar can be as addictive as certain drugs (for example, cocaine) and withdrawal symptoms have also been observed to be similar.

Why is sugar so dangerous?

The sweet seduction of sugar can literally break your heart and negatively impact every organ in your body. Too much sugar can increase your risk of heart disease, type 2 diabetes, kidney disease, cancer, non-alcoholic fatty liver disease, rheumatoid arthritis, worsening joint pain, obesity, impotence, and depression.

What about your external appearance? Sugar can ruin your teeth and accelerate the aging of your skin with more wrinkles and sagging. Besides aging your skin, it increases your risk of developing acne. Finally, sugar can weaken your immune system, making you more vulnerable to illness. Having a weakened immune system is especially relevant now during the COVID-19 pandemic; we each need an optimally performing immune system to combat potential infection.

Let's be proactive! Dining out is here to stay, so we must do our homework and be mindful of how much sugar we consume in a day. I've made your homework a little easier by providing you with my assessment of the best and worst food options, based on the sugar content, at typical restaurant chains.

Before you can discern what is good versus bad regarding sugar consumption, you must know the maximum daily allowance for sugar. The American Heart Association recommends no more than 6 teaspoons or 24 grams of sugar for women and no more than 9 teaspoons or 36 grams of sugar for men. Keep in mind: 4 grams of sugar = 1 teaspoon of sugar. The average American consumes 77 grams or approximately 19 teaspoons of sugar per day, which far exceeds the recommended amount.

My recommendations for best eats in this book are based on the Mediterranean way of eating from the 1950s and 1960s in Spain, Italy, and Greece. It is the most researched diet, and there is solid data that proves its health benefits.

This diet has been shown to help lower blood pressure, cholesterol, heart disease, certain cancer risks, and dementia. So, what are Mediterranean foods? They are predominately plant-based, with the diet focusing on a daily consumption of vegetables, fruits, whole grains, beans, legumes, nuts, seeds, and olive oil.

Certain animal products are allowed in moderation, with a preference for seafood and occasional poultry. It is important to note that red meat and added sugars from non-fruit sources are rarely consumed.

Therefore, my "Best Eats" suggestions in this book will be plant-based foods, fish, and poultry. Red meat and processed meat are excluded.

The International Agency for Research on Cancer, a division of the World Health Organization, has classified processed meats like hot dogs, ham, bacon, sausage, pepperoni, corned beef, and pastrami as Group 1 carcinogens. Group 1 means there is sufficient evidence to link processed meats to cancer. Red meat has been classified as a Group 2A carcinogen, which means that there is some evidence suggesting a link to cancer.

In addition to avoiding processed meats and red meats when dining out, you need to be aware of specific red flag words that indicate a meal is high in calories and added fat.

These red flag words and ingredients include: creamy, buttery, gravy, breaded, stuffed, smothered, au gratin, parmesan, fried, sauces, sauced, cheese sauce, scalloped, au fromage, a la mode, deep-fried, battered, aioli, béarnaise, bisque, confit, carbonara, crunchy, en croute, fritters, golden, hollandaise (made with butter, egg yolks, and lemon juice), pan-fried (depending on what it is fried in), refried (beans mashed and then fried in lard), roux (a mixture of flour and fat—butter, drippings, or pork or beef fat), sautéed (depending on what is used), scalloped (usually potatoes cooked in cream and butter, topped with cheese), scampi (shrimp cooked in butter sauce and garlic), tempura (a Japanese version of batter-dipped and deep-fried), white sauce, and cream sauce.

Tips for Dining Out

Lastly, I want to share some tips to make dining out a healthy—but still tasty—experience. Besides choosing food options low in sugar, these tips can also help guide you in choosing the healthiest dining experience.

1. Use the HappyCow app to find healthier restaurants in your zip code.

2. Look at the nutrition facts before dining out. Ask how the dish was prepared and what ingredients were used. Perhaps they can prepare it the way you like it.

3. Ask if you can substitute fries with a baked potato or a baked sweet potato.

4. Ask if they can grill or broil the food instead of frying it.

5. Ask if they can increase the serving of vegetables with your meal. Typically, the 'servings' of vegetables are simply a bit of decoration to add color.

6. Ask the waiter to box up half of your meal before bringing it to the table. So often, we are compelled to eat everything on our plates, which is especially troublesome since most restaurants typically serve two to three times more food than listed on the food label.

7. Consider ordering two appetizers vs. one entrée meal—it is typically less food, but it can still fill you up.

8. Always order a big salad first. Eating a salad before the entrée will supply your body with more nutrients and, moreover, fewer overall calories. Be careful about what you add to your salad. Leave off the bacon, ham, cheese, croutons, and meats. Always get your salad dressing on the side; otherwise, the salad may be drenched in it.

9. Order seafood. When I looked at the chain restaurants, seafood restaurants like Red Lobster and Bone Fish Grill had far more healthy options with lower sodium, lower sugar, and lower fat.

10. Drink a glass of water before your meal to help decrease your overall calorie intake.

11. Consider bringing your own homemade salad dressing.

12. Ideally, pass on the bread basket and, at the very least, ask for 100% whole grain bread.

13. For dessert, try some sorbet or a piece of dark chocolate instead of high-sugar menu options.

Now let's look at some standard chain restaurants and identify the healthiest and unhealthiest choices based on the amount of sugar in each dish.

Note: Drinks, sweets, breakfast, and bakery items are not included on these lists.

Commit to memory the added sugar content of common beverages. For example:

1. Unsweetened tea: 0 grams

2. Sweetened tea: 29 grams or 7 teaspoons

3. Regular soda: 37 grams or 9 teaspoons

4. Lemonade: 43 grams or 10 teaspoons

5. Fruit drinks: 59 grams or 14 teaspoons

All these beverages, with the exception of unsweetened tea, exceed a woman's daily sugar allowance, which is 6 teaspoons. *In addition*, don't forget to add your sugar intake from both food *and* beverages to get your total daily consumption. I guarantee that you will be appalled at how much sugar you consume in a day.

All fried foods are automatically placed in the Worst Eats category.

DISCLAIMER:
Nutrition facts in this book may vary depending on the source.
Nutrition facts are included in the "Endnotes" section starting on page 37.

Applebee's

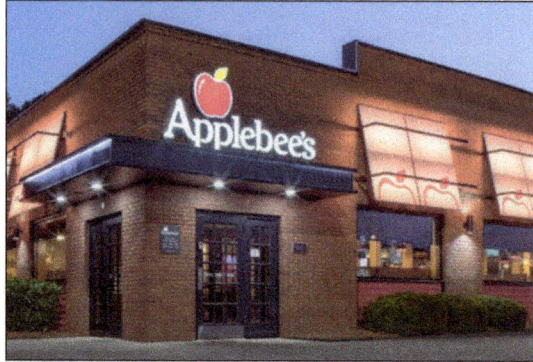

BEST EATS[1]

DISH	SUGAR (GRAMS)
Chicken Breast Burger	0
Broccoli (Steamed)	2
Garlicky Green Beans	2
Blackened Cajun Salmon	4
Grilled Chicken Breast	4
Loaded Baked Potato	4
Bourbon Street Chicken + Shrimp	6
Southwest Chicken Bowl	6
Text-Mex Shrimp Bowl	6
Chipotle Lime Chicken Quesadilla	7

WORST EATS

DISH	SUGAR (GRAMS)
Honey Pepper Boneless Wings	51
Sweet Asian Chile Boneless Wings	46
4 Cheese Mac + Cheese with Honey Peppers Chicken Tenders	41
Honey Barbecue Boneless Wings	39
Oriental Grilled Chicken Salad Wrap	37
Double Crunch Shrimp	30

Consuming a diet high in sugar and fat leads to leptin resistance. Leptin is a critical hormone that controls your hunger and tells you to stop eating. If leptin is not functioning, that can lead to uncontrollable eating and obesity.[2]

MAXIMUM DAILY ALLOWANCE FOR SUGAR
Male: 36 grams or 9 teaspoons
Female: 24 grams or 6 teaspoons

Bonefish Grill

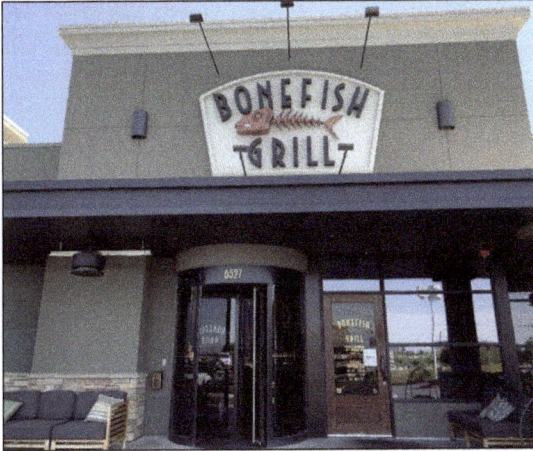

BEST EATS[3]

DISH	SUGAR (GRAMS)
Any grilled fish	0
George Bank Scallops and Shrimp or Scallops and Shrimp Skewer	0
Wood Grilled Chicken	0
Cod Imperial	2
Pecan Parmesan Crusted Rainbow Trout	2
Lily's Chicken	3

WORST EATS

DISH	SUGAR (GRAMS)
Mussels Josephine	25
Ahi Tuna Poke	23
Tuna Poke Bowl	22
Bang Bang Shrimp Tacos (Fried)	19–20
Bonefish Signature Pasta, Cajun Cream plain, with chicken, shrimp or salmon	18
Cod Fish + Chips (Fried)	13
Blackened Baja Fish Tacos	12

Just one 16-ounce can of Coca-Cola supplies your body with 52 grams of added sugar, according to the Coca-Cola Company. This amount is two times the maximum daily amount for women and 1.5 times the daily amount for men.[4]

MAXIMUM DAILY ALLOWANCE FOR SUGAR
Male: 36 grams or 9 teaspoons
Female: 24 grams or 6 teaspoons

Boston Market

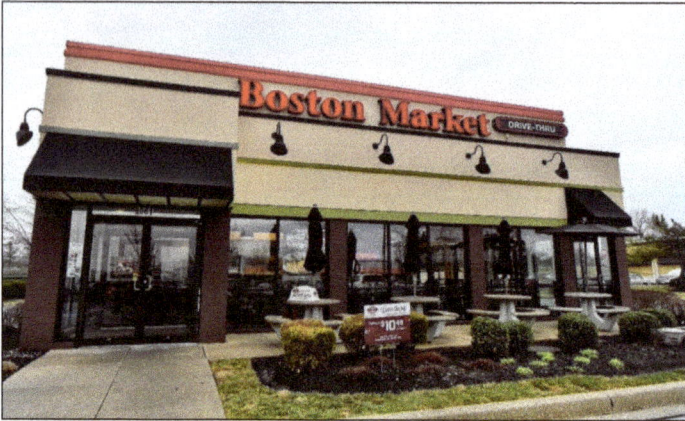

BEST EATS[5]

DISH	SUGAR (GRAMS)
Turkey Breast	0
Rotisserie Chicken (White meat)	0–1
Sesame Chicken, White or Dark Meat	0–1
Rotisserie Chicken (Dark meat)	< 1
Garlic Dill New Potatoes	2
Roasted Garlic and Herb Chicken, White or Dark Meat	2–3
Steamed Broccoli or Steamed Veggies	2–3
Fresh Vegetable Stuffing	5

WORST EATS

DISH	SUGAR (GRAMS)
Sweet Potato Casserole	56
Cinnamon Apples	44
Macaroni + Cheese	10
Sweet Corn	10
Turkey Pot Pie / Rotisserie Chicken Pot Pie	10

People who consume 17–21% of their daily calories from sugar have a 38% greater risk of dying from heart disease.[6]

MAXIMUM DAILY ALLOWANCE FOR SUGAR
Male: 36 grams or 9 teaspoons
Female: 24 grams or 6 teaspoons

BJ's Restaurant

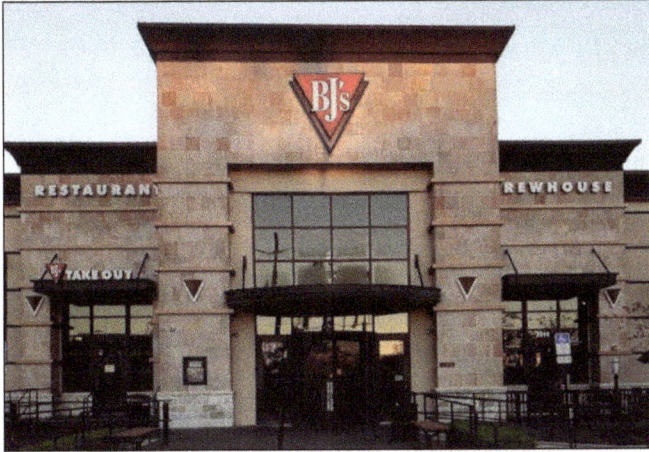

BEST EATS[7]

DISH	SUGAR (GRAMS)
Peruvian Quinoa Bowl with Chicken, Salmon, Shrimp or Vegetarian	5–6
Cajun Grilled Shrimp Tacos	7
Flame-Broiled Mahi-Mahi Tacos	7
Fresh Atlantic Salmon, Flame-Broiled or Blackened	7
Moroccan Chicken	7

WORST EATS

DISH	SUGAR (GRAMS)
Honey Crisp Chicken Salad	36
Kale + Roasted Brussel Sprouts Salad with Blackened Chicken, Salmon, Cajun Shrimp, Flame-Broiled Salmon, or Grilled Chicken	34
Barbeque Chicken Chopped Salad	29
Jumbo Spaghetti + Meatballs	28
Seared Ahi Salad	25
Spicy Peanut Chicken with Soba Noodles	23
Turkey Burger	23

Diets high in sugar can increase insulin resistance, and insulin resistance can increase your risk of cancer, especially breast, prostate, and colon cancer.[8]

There is a positive association between eating too much sugar and obesity. In fact, one daily soda amounts to 32 pounds of sugar per year, which can lead to a 15–25 pound weight gain.[9]

MAXIMUM DAILY ALLOWANCE FOR SUGAR
Male: 36 grams or 9 teaspoons
Female: 24 grams or 6 teaspoons

Cheesecake Factory

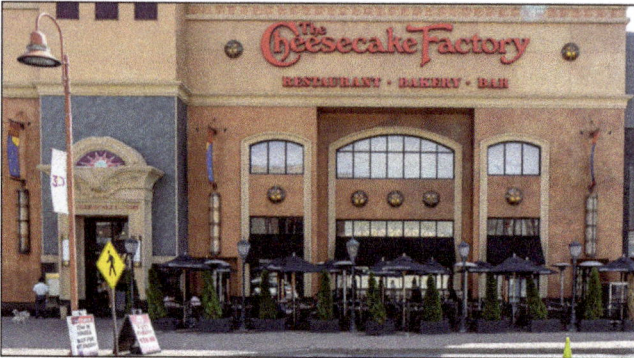

BEST EATS[10]

DISH	SUGAR (GRAMS)
Grilled Asparagus	0
Green Beans	2
Beans and Rice	3
Herb-Crusted Filet of Salmon	4
Margherita Flatbread Pizza	4
Fresh Grilled Salmon	4–6
SkinnyLicious® Tuscan Chicken	5

WORST EATS

DISH	SUGAR (GRAMS)
Crispy Pineapple Chicken and Shrimp	82
Orange Chicken	77
Teriyaki Chicken	75
Barbecue Ranch Chicken Salad	66
Korean Fried Chicken	66
Thai Lettuce Wraps	64-69
Chinese or Thai Chicken Salad	62-63
Spicy Cashew Chicken	62
Jamaican Black Pepper Shrimp/Chicken	60
Island Style Ahi Poke Bowl with Kale-Cashew Salad	54
Carolina Grilled Salmon	42
Chicken Katsu	40

Consumption of too much sugar is associated with negative psychological effects, such as depression.[11]

The most visible effects of the hazards of sugar can be seen in your skin. Sugar disrupts the collagen molecules, causing the skin to lose its elasticity resulting in increased wrinkles and sagging skin.[12]

MAXIMUM DAILY ALLOWANCE FOR SUGAR
Male: 36 grams or 9 teaspoons
Female: 24 grams or 6 teaspoons

Chick-fil-A

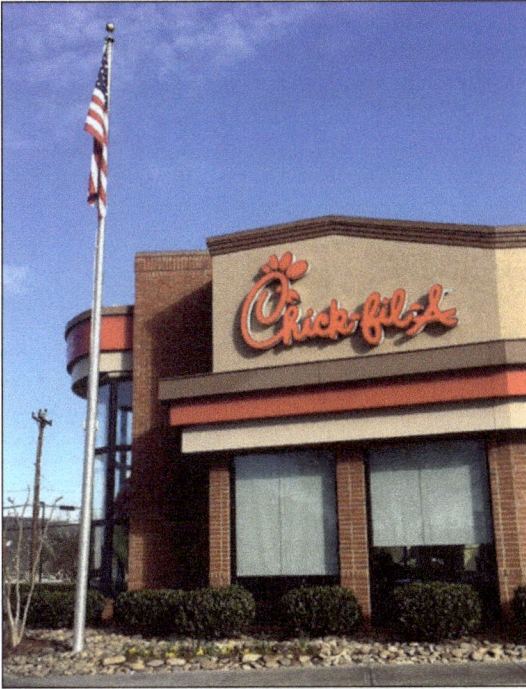

BEST EATS[13]

DISH	SUGAR (GRAMS)
Grilled Nuggets	1
Chick-fil-A Cool Wrap (Grilled)	2
Kale Crunch Salad Side or Side Salad	3

WORST EATS

DISH	SUGAR (GRAMS)
Greek Yogurt Parfait	26
Market Salad	26
Chick-fil-A Grilled Club Sandwich	11

A daily intake of sugar-sweetened drinks was associated with a greater than 50% increased risk of non-alcoholic fatty liver disease.[14]

MAXIMUM DAILY ALLOWANCE FOR SUGAR
Male: 36 grams or 9 teaspoons
Female: 24 grams or 6 teaspoons

Chili's

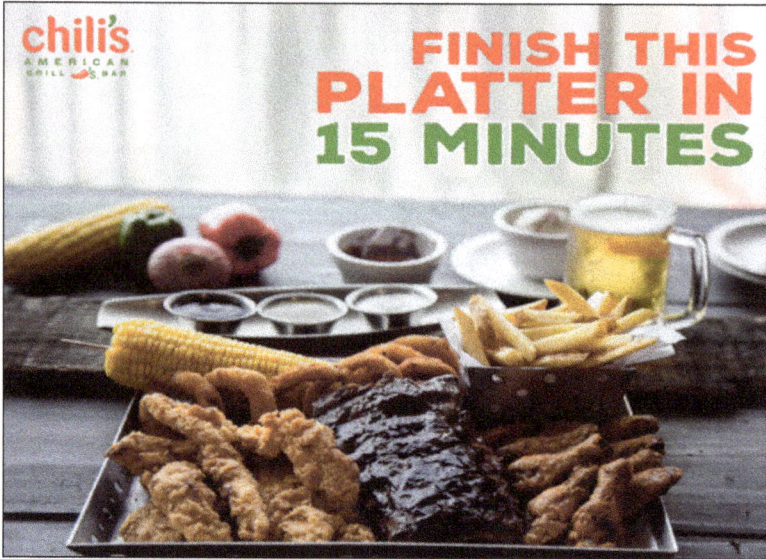

BEST EATS[15]

DISH	SUGAR (GRAMS)
Grilled Chicken Fajitas (Mix & Match 1 Portion)	0
Seared Shrimp (Mix & Match 1 Portion)	0
Black Bean Patty	2
Black Beans + Mexican Rice	3
Guiltless Grill Ancho Salmon	5

WORST EATS

DISH	SUGAR (GRAMS)
Crispy Honey Chipotle + Waffles	128
Crispy Honey Chipotle Crispers	66
Bone-in Wings Honey Chipotle or Boneless Wings Honey Chipotle	53
Crispy Mango Habanero Crispers	37
Boneless Wings - House BBQ	30
Boneless Wings Mango Habanero	25

Too much sugar leads to cavities and poor oral health.[16]

MAXIMUM DAILY ALLOWANCE FOR SUGAR
Male: 36 grams or 9 teaspoons
Female: 24 grams or 6 teaspoons

Cracker Barrel

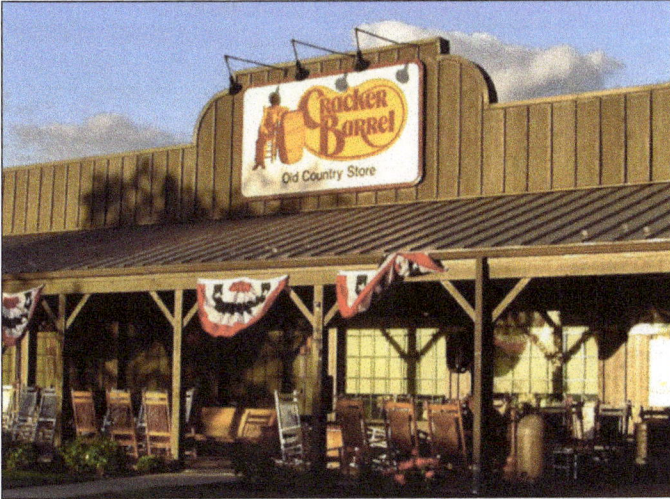

BEST EATS[17]

DISH	SUGAR (GRAMS)
Lemon Pepper Grilled Rainbow Trout	0
Spicy Grilled Catfish	0
Broccoli Cheddar Chicken	1
Grilled Chicken Tenders	4
Bowl of Beans (has meat)	7
Homestyle Grilled Chicken Salad	7

WORST EATS

DISH	SUGAR (GRAMS)
Loaded Baked Sweet Potato	56
Turkey n' Dressing	41
Maple Bacon Grilled Chicken	27
Country Fried Shrimp	15

Too much sugar is associated with an increased risk of dementia.[18]

MAXIMUM DAILY ALLOWANCE FOR SUGAR
Male: 36 grams or 9 teaspoons
Female: 24 grams or 6 teaspoons

Golden Corral

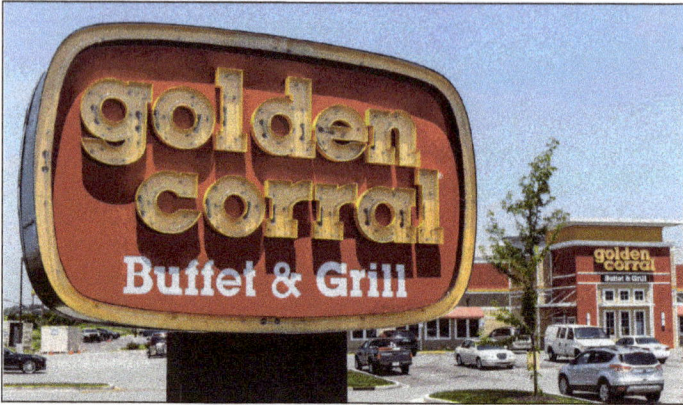

BEST EATS[19]

DISH	SUGAR (GRAMS)
Baked Fish with Lemon Herb Sauce / Piccata Sauce / Florentine	0
Butterfly Shrimp	0
Carved Salmon	0
Carved Turkey (Dark or White)	0
Golden Roasted Chicken / Rotisserie (Dark or White)	0
Smoky Garlic Grilled Shrimp Skewer	0
Chicken Machaca	1
Chicken Piccata	1
Chicken Quesadillas	1
Lemon Herb Chicken	1
Chicken Fajita	2

WORST EATS

DISH	SUGAR (GRAMS)
Honey-Dipped Fried Chicken	321
Korean Style Fried Chicken	120
Chicken + Waffles Bowl	68
Orange Chicken	29
Grilled Hickory Bourbon Chicken	27

Drink more water or sparkling water.
Be proactive! Find out the nutrition facts before going out to a restaurant.

MAXIMUM DAILY ALLOWANCE FOR SUGAR
Male: 36 grams or 9 teaspoons
Female: 24 grams or 6 teaspoons

Jack in the Box

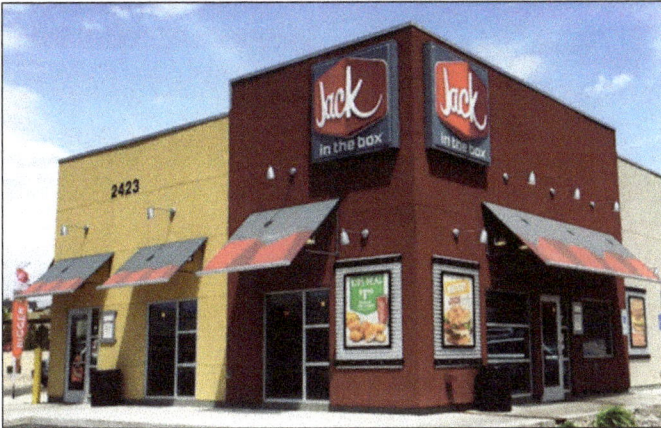

BEST EATS[20]

DISH	SUGAR (GRAMS)
Chicken Fajita with Whole Grain	3
Chicken Strips, Grilled	3
Grilled Sandwich, Turkey without Bacon	4
Grilled Chicken Salad	6
Sourdough Grilled Chicken Club without Bacon	6

WORST EATS

DISH	SUGAR (GRAMS)
Chicken Teriyaki Bowl	36
Chiquita Apple Bites with Carmel	13
Grilled Chicken Strips with Teriyaki Dipping Sauce	12
Any dish with added Barbecue, Teriyaki or Honey Mustard Dipping Sauce	9–10

*Buy plain yogurt and add your fruit instead of buying those sweetened with added sugar.
My favorite brand is Forager Project Organic Plant-based Cashewmilk Yogurt.*

MAXIMUM DAILY ALLOWANCE FOR SUGAR
Male: 36 grams or 9 teaspoons
Female: 24 grams or 6 teaspoons

KFC

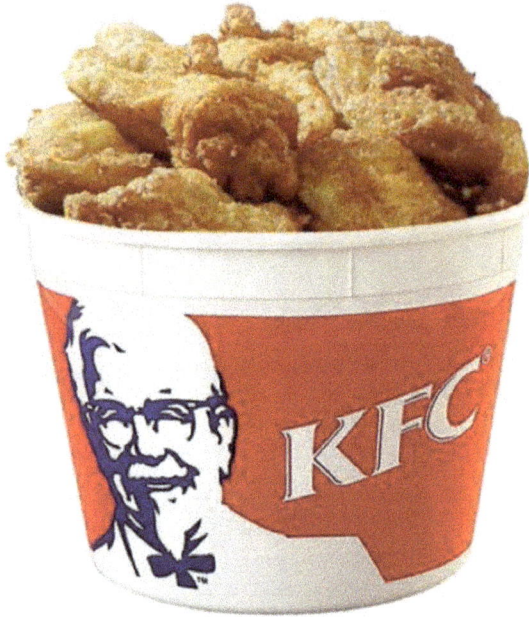

BEST EATS[21]

DISH	SUGAR (GRAMS)
Grilled Breast	0
Grilled Drumstick	0
Grilled Thigh	0
Grilled Wing	0

WORST EATS

DISH	SUGAR (GRAMS)
BBQ Baked Beans	15
KFC Cornbread Muffin	11
Coleslaw	10

For salad dressings, use oil and vinegar or lite vinaigrette. Check out the best-recommended salad dressings for diabetics.[22]

MAXIMUM DAILY ALLOWANCE FOR SUGAR
Male: 36 grams or 9 teaspoons
Female: 24 grams or 6 teaspoons

McDonald's

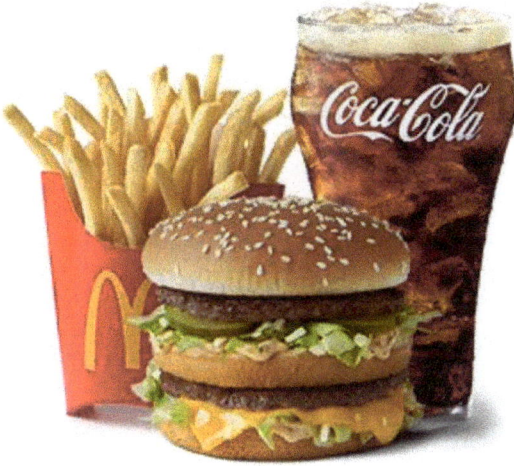

BEST EATS[23]

DISH	SUGAR (GRAMS)
Ranch Snack Wrap®(Grilled)	2
Honey Mustard Snack Wrap® (Grilled)	4
Premium Caesar Salad (w/o chicken)	4
Chipotle BBQ Snack Wrap® (Grilled)	5
Premium Caesar Salad with Grilled Chicken	5
Premium Southwest Salad (without chicken)	6

WORST EATS

DISH	SUGAR (GRAMS)
Barbeque sauce (1 packet)	10
Premium Crispy Chicken Classic Sandwich	10
Sweet and Sour Sauce (1 packet)	10
Honey (1 packet)	11
Premium Crispy Chicken Club Sandwich	11
Premium Crispy Chicken Ranch BLT Sandwich	11
Premium Southwest Salad with Grilled Chicken	11
Southwestern Chipotle Barbeque Sauce (1 packet)	11
Premium Southwest Salad with Crispy Chicken	12

Why not make your own salad dressing? Just Google "3-ingredient salad dressing".[24]

MAXIMUM DAILY ALLOWANCE FOR SUGAR
Male: 36 grams or 9 teaspoons
Female: 24 grams or 6 teaspoons

Olive Garden

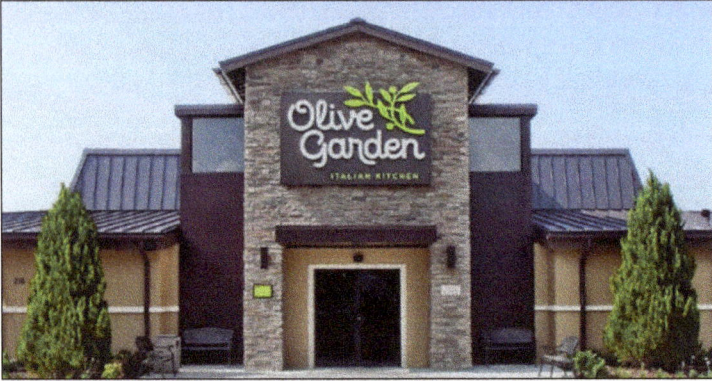

SPAGHETTI WITH MARINARA SAUCE

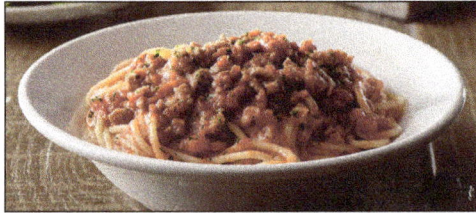

BEST EATS[25]

DISH	SUGAR (GRAMS)
Herbed Grilled Salmon or Herbed Grilled Salmon Coho	3
Salad with Signature Italian Dressing	4
Grilled Chicken Margherita	5
Shrimp Scampi	5
Chicken Scampi	7

WORST EATS

DISH	SUGAR (GRAMS)
Eggplant Parmigiana	23
Giant Cheese-Stuffed Shells	22
Five-Cheese Ziti al Forno	19
Chicken Parmigiana	16
Tour of Italy	12
Lasagna Classico	11

Sugar may taste heavenly, but it is one of the most inflammation-provoking and addictive substances you can put in your body.

MAXIMUM DAILY ALLOWANCE FOR SUGAR
Male: 36 grams or 9 teaspoons
Female: 24 grams or 6 teaspoons

Outback Steakhouse

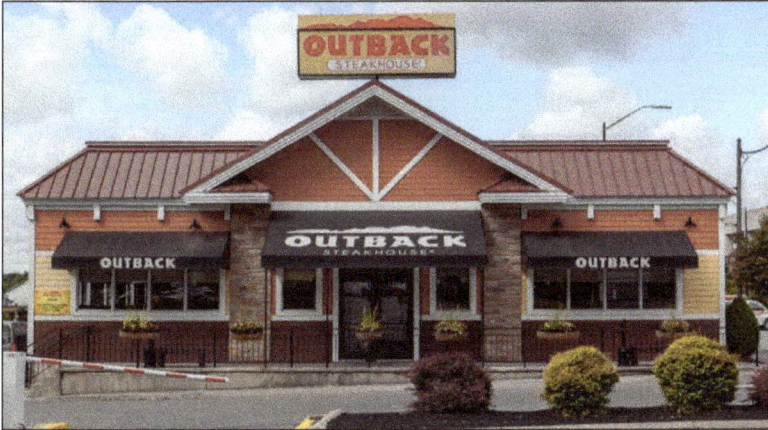

BEST EATS[26]

DISH	SUGAR (GRAMS)
Lobster Tail, 5oz (Steamed or Grilled)	0
Simply Grilled Mahi	0
Queensland Pasta with Chicken or Chicken + Shrimp	< 1
Simply Grilled Halibut	1
Simply Grilled Salmon, 8oz or 10oz	1
Alice Springs Chicken, 5oz	6
Grilled Shrimp	6

WORST EATS

DISH	SUGAR (GRAMS)
Entrée Asian Chicken Salad with Dressing	36
Bloomin' Onion (appetizer)	34
Entrée Asian Salad with Ahi and Dressing	22
Gold Coast Coconut Shrimp (appetizer)	21
House Side Salad with Tangy Tomato Dressing	16
Chicken Tender Platter with Honey Mustard	15
Grilled Chicken on the Barbie	14
Bloomin' Fried Chicken Sandwich	13
Bloomin' Fried Chicken	11

Try Sprouts Reduced Sugar and Sodium Ketchup.
Try Stevia Sweet BBQ Sauce or Organicville Spicy Southwest BBQ Sauce.

MAXIMUM DAILY ALLOWANCE FOR SUGAR
Male: 36 grams or 9 teaspoons
Female: 24 grams or 6 teaspoons

Panda Express

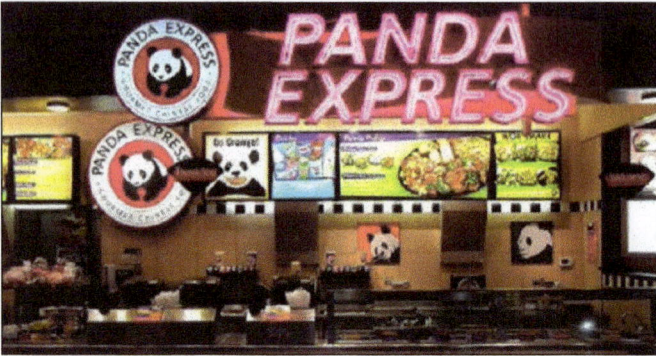

NOTE: ORDERING FROM THE KIDS' MENU CAN BE A HEALTHIER ALTERNATIVE

BEST EATS[27]

DISH	SUGAR (GRAMS)
Brown Steamed Rice	0–1
Chicken Potsticker (appetizer)	2
Super Greens or Super Greens Entrée	2–4
Fried Rice	3
Firecracker Shrimp Entrée	4
Potato Chicken	4
Stringbean Chicken	4
Mushroom Chicken	5

WORST EATS

DISH	SUGAR (GRAMS)
Sweet Fire Chicken Breast	27
Sweet & Sour Chicken Breast	24
Sweet and Sour Sauce	20
Honey Sesame Chicken Breast	19
Orange Chicken	19
Eggplant Tofu	17
Golden Treasure Shrimp	14
Teriyaki Sauce	14
Asian Chicken	10
Teriyaki Chicken	10

For breakfast, cook some steel-cut oatmeal in an Instapot and add some cut-up banana and apple along with some cinnamon. Once done, you will have a bowl of sweet oats with caramelized fruit. There will be no need to add any sugar!

MAXIMUM DAILY ALLOWANCE FOR SUGAR
Male: 36 grams or 9 teaspoons
Female: 24 grams or 6 teaspoons

Panera Bread

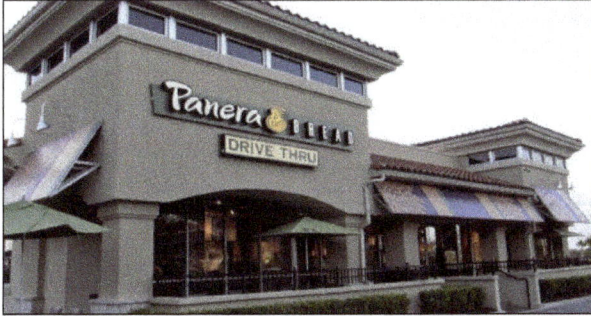

BEST EATS[28]

DISH	SUGAR (GRAMS)
Smoked Chicken (Double Portion)	0
Sliced Turkey (Double Portion)	1
Chipotle Chicken Avocado Melt on Black Pepper Focaccia (1/2)	2
Double Tuna Salad	2
Frontega Chicken Panini on Black Pepper Focaccia (1/2)	3
Tuna Salad on Black Pepper Focaccia (1/2)	3
Turkey on Country Rustic Sourdough (1/2)	3
Mediterranean Veggie on Tomato Basil (1/2)	4
Chipotle Chicken Avocado Melt on Black Pepper Focaccia (Whole)	5
Frontega Chicken Panini on Black Pepper Focaccia (Whole)	6
Tuna Salad on Black Pepper Focaccia (Whole)	6

WORST EATS

DISH	SUGAR (GRAMS)
Vegetarian Autumn Squash Soup Cup to Bowl	22–33
Teriyaki Chicken Broccoli Bowl	25
Fuji Apple with Chicken Entrée Salad	23
Smokehouse Barbecue Chicken on Classic White Miche (Whole)	18
Barbecue Chicken Salad (Entrée)	14
Grilled Mac & Cheese on Classic White Miche (Whole)	14
Classic Grilled Cheese (Whole)	11
Green Goddess Cobb with Chicken Entrée Salad	11
Napa Almond Chicken Salad on Country Rustic Sourdough	11

Did you know the brain MRI of a sugar-addicted person is very similar to that of a cocaine-addicted person?

MAXIMUM DAILY ALLOWANCE FOR SUGAR
Male: 36 grams or 9 teaspoons
Female: 24 grams or 6 teaspoons

Red Lobster

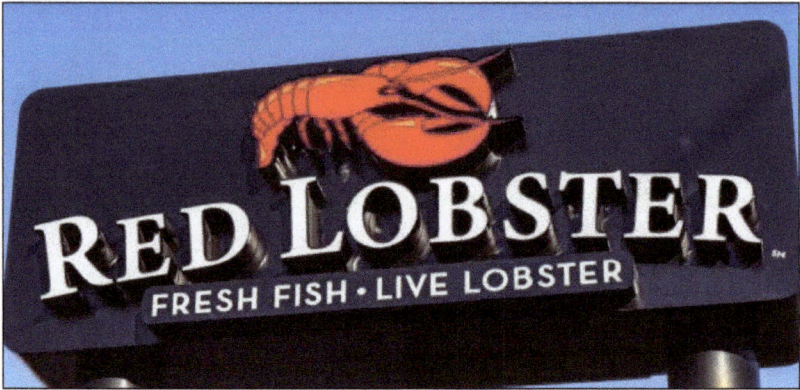

BEST EATS[29]

DISH	SUGAR (GRAMS)
Simply Grilled Atlantic Salmon	0
Simply Grilled Rainbow Trout	0
Wild Caught Snow Crab Legs	0
Quinoa Rice	<1
Simply Grilled Garlic Shrimp Skewers	1
Classic Caesar Salad Plain or with Grilled Chicken or Salmon	3
Salmon New Orleans	3

WORST EATS

DISH	SUGAR (GRAMS)
Kung Pao Noodles with Chicken, Lobster, or Shrimp	89
Nashville Hot Chicken Sandwich	32
Parrot Isle Jumbo Coconut Shrimp	28
Sesame-Soy Salmon Bowl	28
Crab Stuffed Shrimp Rangoon	24
Fish & Chips	22
Crispy Brussels Sprouts	19
Admiral's Feast	16

Aim for zero added sugars!

MAXIMUM DAILY ALLOWANCE FOR SUGAR
Male: 36 grams or 9 teaspoons
Female: 24 grams or 6 teaspoons

Subway

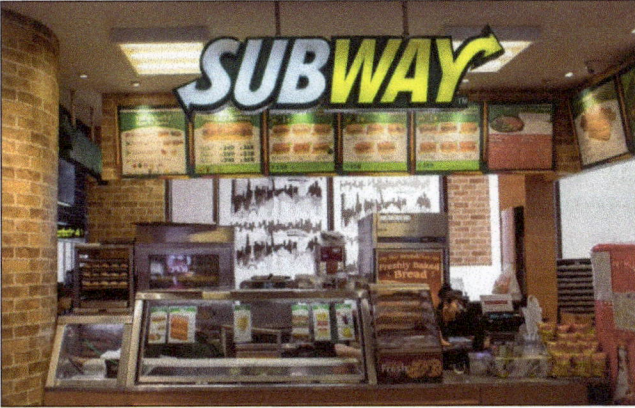

NOTE: IT IS RECOMMENDED TO NOT EAT ANY PROCESSED MEATS

BEST EATS[30]

DISH	SUGAR (GRAMS)
6" Subway Seafood Sensation	4
Veggie Flatizza	5
6" Tuna	5
6" Veggie Delite	5
6" Oven-Roasted Chicken	6
6" Rotisserie-style Chicken	6
6" Turkey Breast	6

WORST EATS

DISH	SUGAR (GRAMS)
Sweet Onion Teriyaki Bowl	22
6" Sweet Teriyaki Chicken on Tomato Basil	14
Chicken Pizziola with Grilled Chicken	10
Any Item with Teriyaki Sauce	8

According to a recent study, diets rich in sugary foods are linked with the development of acne as an adult.[31]

MAXIMUM DAILY ALLOWANCE FOR SUGAR
Male: 36 grams or 9 teaspoons
Female: 24 grams or 6 teaspoons

Taco Bell

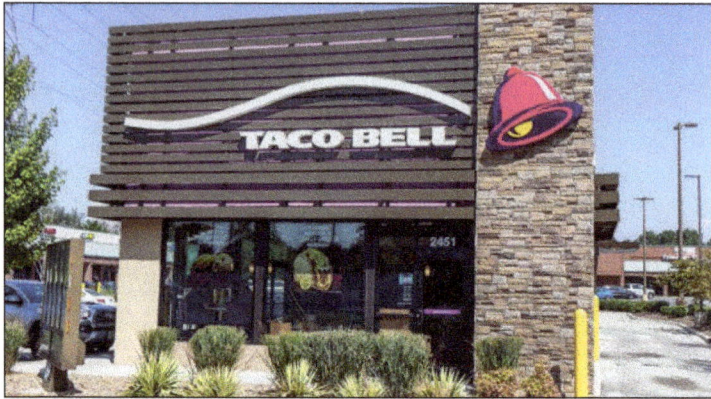

BEST EATS[32]

DISH	SUGAR (GRAMS)
Black Beans & Rice	0
Soft Taco Chicken	1
Cantina Crispy Melt Taco Chicken	2
Cantina Crispy Melt Taco with Black Beans	2
Soft Taco Supreme	2
Power Veggie Bowl	3
Black Bean Chalupa	4
Chalupa Supreme Chicken	4

WORST EATS

DISH	SUGAR (GRAMS)
Black Bean Crunchwrap Supreme	6
Crunchwrap Supreme	6

Make your own soda! Add ¼ cup of your favorite 100% juice and ¾ cup of sparkling water. With this beverage, you have the fizz-fizz without all the sugar, artificial flavoring, and calories.

MAXIMUM DAILY ALLOWANCE FOR SUGAR
Male: 36 grams or 9 teaspoons
Female: 24 grams or 6 teaspoons

Wendy's

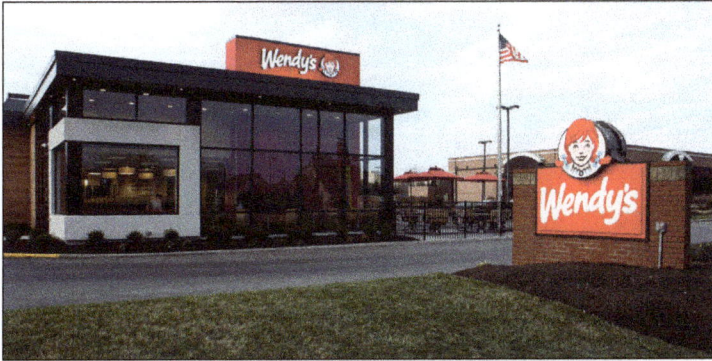

BEST ENTRÉES (EATS)[33]

DISH	SUGAR (GRAMS)
Grilled Chicken Wrap	3
Plain Baked Potato	3
Summer Berry Burst Fruit Cup	3
Baked Potato with Sour Cream and Chives	4
Southwest Avocado Chicken Salad without Bacon – 1/2 salad	4
Apple Bites	7
Southwest Avocado Chicken Salad without Bacon – full salad	7

WORST EATS

DISH	SUGAR (GRAMS)
Apple Pecan Chicken Salad	40
Berry Burst Chicken Salad	29
Taco Salad	18
Cheese Baked Potato	14

Check out **Women's Health Magazine** *for the best low-sugar cereals of 2021.*[34]

MAXIMUM DAILY ALLOWANCE FOR SUGAR
Male: 36 grams or 9 teaspoons
Female: 24 grams or 6 teaspoons

Yard House

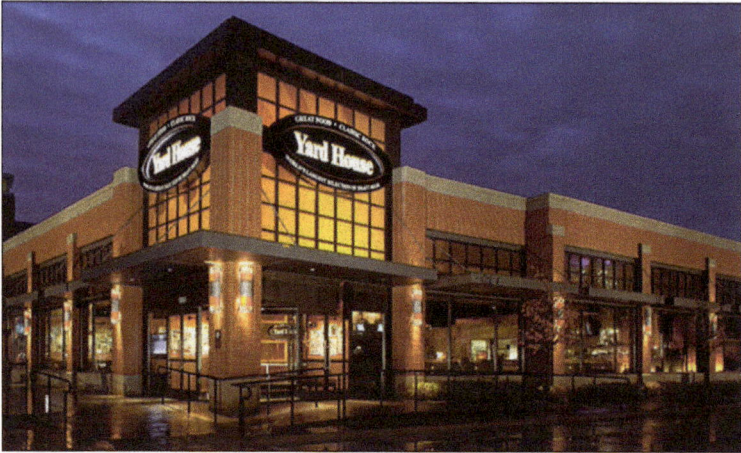

BEST EATS[35]

DISH	SUGAR (GRAMS)
Baja Fish Tacos	1
Blackened Swordfish Tacos	1
Chicken Tinga Tacos	2
Cilantro Lime Grilled Shrimp	3.7
Vodka Shrimp Pasta	4.7
Porcini Crusted Halibut	5.8
Turkey Burger	6

WORST EATS

DISH	SUGAR (GRAMS)
Orange Peel Chicken	66
Coconut Shrimp (Appetizer)	64
Chicken Lettuce Wraps with Sweet Chili Sauce	46
Sweet Potato Fries (Snack)	42
Boneless Firecracker Wings	40
Entrée Barbecue Chicken Salad	40
Fresh Island Macadamia Nut Crusted Fish	34
Fresh Island Blackened Fish or Grilled Fish	23/22
Chicken Rice Bowl	22
Ginger-Crusted Norwegian Salmon	20

Consumption of sugar-sweetened beverages is associated with a 30% higher risk of developing Type 2 Diabetes.[36]

MAXIMUM DAILY ALLOWANCE FOR SUGAR
Male: 36 grams or 9 teaspoons
Female: 24 grams or 6 teaspoons

About Trina Wiggins, MD

Dr. Trina Wiggins is a board-certified pediatrician in Las Vegas, Nevada. She attended Stanford University, where she received a BA degree in human biology and was the first African American on Stanford Women's Gymnastics Team. After graduating from Stanford University, she attended medical school at Washington University School of Medicine in St. Louis, Missouri, and completed her internship and residency at Cardinal Glennon Children's Hospital. She has worked in both the public and private sectors. Most recently, she has volunteered with Volunteers in Medicine for over ten years.

In addition to being a pediatrician, Dr. Trina competes in fitness and dance competitions. She has competed in over fifty shows over the past nineteen years, with many top-place finishes. In 2011, she placed first in the Fitness America Classic. In 2018, she competed in the Nevada State Senior Olympics and received a gold medal. Furthermore, she was named the AAU North American Bodybuilding and Fitness 2019 Athlete of the Year.

On December 5, 2021, she competed in the World Fitness Forum and received first place. She is currently the president of the Stanford Club of Southern Nevada, and from 2015–2016 she served as the president of the Stanford National Black Alumni Association.

In June 2020, she published her first book, entitled *KISS: Keep It Short and Simple for a Healthy, Sustainable Lifestyle*. She bundled all her knowledge as a physician, former collegiate athlete, and fitness professional to create the ultimate guide for living a healthy yet simple lifestyle. Be on the watch for the 2nd edition of KISS in 2022. She is married to Dr. Carl Allen and has three children and one granddaughter. Her twin sons graduated from Stanford University in June 2017, and her daughter is a practicing attorney in Houston, Texas. Her granddaughter is currently in the tenth grade.

Endnotes

1. Applebee's Menu Nutrition Facts, Accessed April 2022, https://www.applebees.com/en/nutrition/info.

2. Alexandra Shapiro, "Prevention and reversal of diet-induced leptin resistance with a sugar-free diet despite high fat content," August 2011, https://pubmed.ncbi.nlm.nih.gov /21418711/

3. Menu Label Report: Bonefish Grill Nutrition Information, Accessed April 2022, https://az727285.vo.msecnd.net /menu/bonefishgrill_nutritional_information.pdf.

4. "How much sugar is in Coca-Cola," The Coca-Cola Company, Accessed April 2022, https://www.coca -colacompany.com/faqs/how-much-sugar-is-in-coca -cola#:~:text=in%2Dcoca%2Dcola-,There%20are%20 39%20grams%20of%20sugar%20in%20a%2012%20 oz,less%20sugar%20and%20fewer%20calories.

5. Boston Market Nutrition Facts & Calorie Information, Nutrition-Charts.com, Updated 2021, https://www.nutrition-charts.com /boston-market-nutrition-facts-calorie-information/

6. Ndumele, https://www.hopkinsmedicine.org/health /wellness-and-prevention/obesity-sugar-and-heart-health

7. "BJ's Interactive Nutrition Menu," NutritionIX, Updated August 29, 2019, http://www.nutritionix.com/bjs-restaurants/menu/premium?desktop.

8. Danielle Underferth, "Sugar, insulin resistance and cancer: What's the link?," June 21, 2021, https://www.mdanderson.org/cancerwise/sugar--insulin-resistance-and-cancer--what-is-the-link.h00-159461634.html.

9. R. Alexander Bentley, "U.S. obesity as delayed effect of excess sugar," ScienceDirect Economics & Human Biology Volume 36, January 2020, https://www.sciencedirect.com/science/article/pii/S1570677X19301364.

10. The Cheesecake Factory Nutritional Guide, The Cheesecake Factory, Accessed April 2022, https://www.thecheesecakefactory.com/assets/pdf/Nutritional_Guide.pdf.

11. Anika Knüppel, Martin J. Shipley, Clare H. Llewellyn, and Eric J. Brunner, "Sugar intake from sweet food and beverages, common mental disorder and depression: prospective findings from the Whitehall II study," National Library of Medicine Scientific Reports, July 27, 2017, https://www.ncbi.nlm.nih.gov/pmc/articles/PMC5532289/.

12. F. William Danby, MD, "Nutrition and Aging Skin: Sugar and Glycation Abstract," Clinics in Dermatology, July 1, 2010, https://www.cidjournal.com/article/S0738-081X(10)00042-8/pdf.

13. Nutrition & Allergens, Chick-fil-a, Accessed April 2022, https://www.chick-fil-a.com/nutrition-allergens.

14. Jiantao Ma, Caroline S Fox, Paul F Jacques, Elizabeth K Speliotes, Udo Hoffmann, Caren E Smith, Edward Saltzman, Nicola M McKeown, "Sugar-sweetened beverage, diet soda, and fatty liver disease in the Framingham Heart Study cohorts Abstract," August 2015, https://pubmed.ncbi.nlm.nih.gov/26055949/.

15. Chili's Nutrition, Accessed April 2022, https://brinker-chilis .cdn.prismic.io/brinker-chilis/a9bf592a-a1a3-4d99-b183 -700b5bfe5188_Chilis-Nutrition-Menu-Generic.pdf.

16. "Sugars and dental caries," World Health Organization, Accessed April 2022, https://www.who.int/news-room /fact-sheets/detail/sugars-and-dental-caries.

17. "Nutrition Facts N' Figures," Crackel Barrel Restaurants, Accessed April 14, 2022, https://prod-cbdigitalstore.azurefd .net/-/media/Project/cb-brandsite/brandsite/pdfs/Nutrition Guide.pdf?rev=adc5fe1642634da9b88dcff484992505&has h=28C9B3E718C9A283C5726FACC1D4B9FC.

18. Paul K. Crane, M.D., M.P.H., Rod Walker, M.S., Rebecca A. Hubbard, Ph.D., Ge Li, M.D., Ph.D., David M. Nathan, M.D., Hui Zheng, Ph.D., Sebastien Haneuse, Ph.D., Suzanne Craft, Ph.D., Thomas J. Montine, M.D., Ph.D., Steven E. Kahn, M.B., Ch.B., Wayne McCormick, M.D., M.P.H., Susan M. McCurry, Ph.D., James D. Bowen, M.D., and Eric B. Larson, M.D., M.P.H, "Glucose Levels and Risk of Dementia," National Library of Medicine, Accessed April 14, 2022, https://www.ncbi.nlm.nih .gov/pmc/articles/PMC3955123/.

19. "Nutrition Facts," Golden Corral, Accessed April 14, 2022, https://www.goldencorral.com/nutrition/.

20. Nutrition Facts, Jack in the Box, Accessed April 2022, http://static.jackinthebox.com/pdfs/nutritional_brochure.pdf

21. Interactive Nutrition Menu, Kentucky Fried Chicken, January 10, 2022, https://www.kfc.com/full-nutrition-guide.

22. Christina Manian, RDN, "The Best Salad Dressings for People with Diabetes," Taste of Home, January 19, 2021, https://www.tasteofhome.com/collection/the-best-salad -dressings-for-people-with-diabetes/.

23. McDonald's USA Nutrition Facts for Popular Menu Items, McDonalds. Accessed April 2022, http://nutrition.mcdonalds .com/nutrition1/nutritionfacts.pdf.

24. 8 Simple and Healthy Salad Dressings, Healthline, Accessed April 2022, www.healthline.com/nutrition/healthy -salad-dressing.

25. Olive Garden Nutrition Information, Olive Garden, March 21, 2022, https://media.olivegarden.com/en_us/pdf/olive _garden_nutrition.pdf.

26. Outback Steakhouse Nutrition Information, Outback Steakhouse, Updated March 2022, https://outback.blob .core.windows.net/content/images/OBS_Full_Nutrition _Information_Core_Menu_Items.pdf.

27. Nutrition & Allergen Information, Panda Express, Accessed April 2022, https://www.pandaexpress.com /nutritioninformation.

28. Panera Bread Menu, Panera Bread, Accessed March 2022, https://www.panerabread.com/content/dam/panerabread/ documents/nutrition/Panera-Nutrition.pdf.

29. Nutrition and Allergy Portal, Red Lobster, Accessed April 2022: https://www.redlobster.com/nutrition-tools.

30. Subway U.S. Nutrition Information, Subway, November 2021, https://www.subway.com/-/media/USA/Documents /Nutrition/US_Nutrition_Values.PDF.

31. Laetitia Penso, MSc; Mathilde Touvier, PhD; Mélanie Desch asaux, PhD, "Association Between Adult Acne and Dietary Behaviors," June 10, 2020, https://jamanetwork.com /journals/jamadermatology/fullarticle/2767075.

32. Full Nutrition Info, Taco Bell, https://www.tacobell.com /nutrition/info. Updated April 5, 2022.

33. Wendy's Nutrition Facts & Calorie Information: Wendy's Menu Nutritional Guide: Food Data & Values, Nutrition -Charts.com, Updated 2021, https://order.wendys.com /categories?site=menu, https://www.nutrition-charts.com /wendys-nutrition-facts-calorie-information/

34. Brittney Loggins, "The 10 Best Low-Sugar Cereal Options Of 2022, According To Nutritionists," Women's Health,

June 7, 2021, https://www.womenshealthmag.com/food/g36599418/low-sugar-cereal/.

35. Yard House Restaurants Nutritional Information, Yard House, Updated October 27, 2014, https://media.yardhouse.com/test/en_us/pdf/yard_house_nutrition.pdf#:~:text=Yard%20House%20Restaurants%20Nutritional%20Information%20Snacks%20Total%20Calories,Carbs%20(g)%20Fiber%20(g)%20Sugars%20(g)%20Protein%20(g).

36. Association between sugar-sweetened beverages and type 2 diabetes: A meta-analysis, Meng Wang, Min Yu, Le Fang, Ru-Ying Hu, National Library of Medicine, December 2, 2014, https://www.ncbi.nlm.nih.gov/pmc/articles/PMC4420570/.

Connect and Share

If you enjoyed *Sugar Seduction* and believe it can help others, please share this book by purchasing copies for others and be sure to leave a review on amazon.com or barnesandnoble.com.

Connect with Dr. Trina Wiggins:
Website: www.trinawiggins.com
Instagram: trina.r.wigginsmd
Facebook: trinawigginsmd
Twitter: trinawiggins123
LinkedIn: https://www.linkedin.com/in/trina-wiggins

www.ingramcontent.com/pod-product-compliance
Lightning Source LLC
Chambersburg PA
CBHW052124030426
42335CB00025B/3105